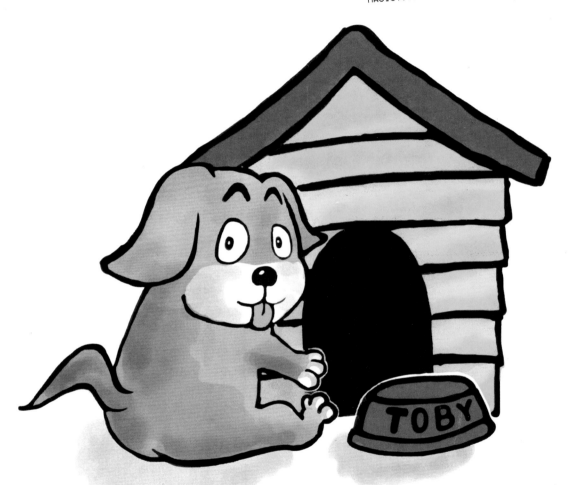

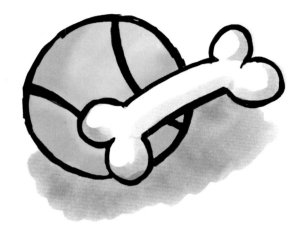

Written and Illustrated by Michale Ok, MD

ISBN-13: 978-0692899854 (Yaeley Bookworks)
ISBN-10: 0692899855

Parents Please Read!

Dear parents, my name is Dr. Michale Ok. Preparing for your child's surgery can be a stressful time for the whole family. There are so many questions that parents can have about anesthesia, surgery and what the day of surgery will be like for their child. As a practicing pediatric anesthesiologist, I find that parents are often given very little information about what to expect on the day of surgery. This leads to poor parent-child communication and on the morning of surgery this lack of communication can manifest in many negative ways. Some parents attempt to talk to their children beforehand but many feel ill-equipped to start that discussion. That is why I decided to write this storybook. This story will walk you through what a typical experience of a healthy child maybe for elective surgery. This storybook is not intended to be a complete guide through anesthesia and surgery but I hope that it will serve as a tool to start conversations with your child.

I want to mention to parents that your child's experience may vary significantly from Toby's story according to both your child's medical condition and surgery. Therefore, please discuss with your children that their experience will not be exactly like Toby's. Setting proper expectations for your children at home will help them have a much more pleasant experience at the hospital. Your anesthesiologist will assess each patient and will always plan his or her anesthetic in the way that is safest for your child. The anesthetic plan will be determined at the sole discretion of your anesthesiologist on the day of surgery.

Since information about anesthesia and surgery can be anxiety provoking, I highly recommend that parents read the contents of this book prior to reading it to their children.

By reading this disclaimer, you acknowledge that I will not be medically or legally liable for any real or perceived negative consequences of reading this book to your child.

General Tips

1. Always thoroughly review and follow your pre-operative instructions given by your physician and hospital.
2. Please keep in mind that different surgeries will have different preparation instructions. If you have questions, please contact your physician prior to surgery. Do not assume anything.
3. On the morning of surgery, there will be specific instructions for not eating or drinking prior to surgery. These are called NPO guidelines. NPO violations are potentially life threatening if not known before anesthesia and will most likely lead to significant delay or even cancelation of your child's surgery.
4. Most surgeries will require an intravenous (IV) line placement. Your anesthesiologist will decide based on your child's medical history whether this will be placed before or after general anesthesia.
5. If your child is developing a respiratory infection prior to surgery, please contact your physician because this may significantly increase your child's risk of anesthesia.
6. Take a deep breath. Your anesthesiologist and surgeon are highly trained, highly skilled physicians who have trained extensively for pediatric care.

Dedication

To my daughter Lydia,

I wrote this book while I was thinking of you. You are my inspiration and perfect gift from the Lord. I love you and thank you for blessing your mother and I everyday.

To my wife Yedeun,

Without your constant encouragement and support, I would have never started this journey of writing my own book. Thank you for constantly challenging me to be better tomorrow than I was today. I love you with all my heart.

To my parents,

Your never-ending love has made me who I am today. I can never thank you enough for your sacrifice. I love you and pray for you every day.

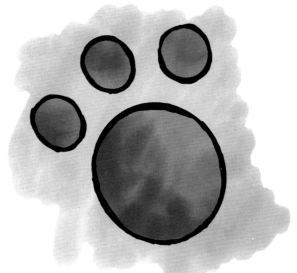

Poor Toby has a boo boo
His front paw hurts a lot
He shows Mom just where it aches
It's in one little spot

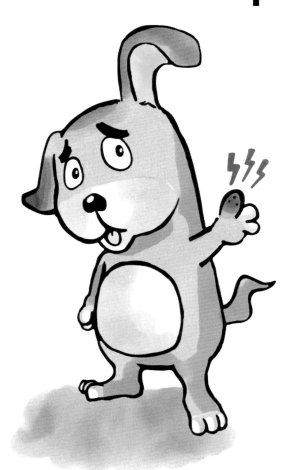

Toby does not want to play
Not even with his ball
He won't fetch a stick or toy
He will not play at all

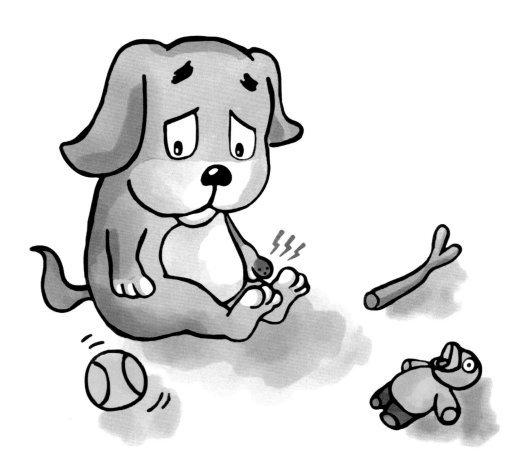

Toby will have surgery
To help him to get well
He should rest at home for now
And soon he will feel swell

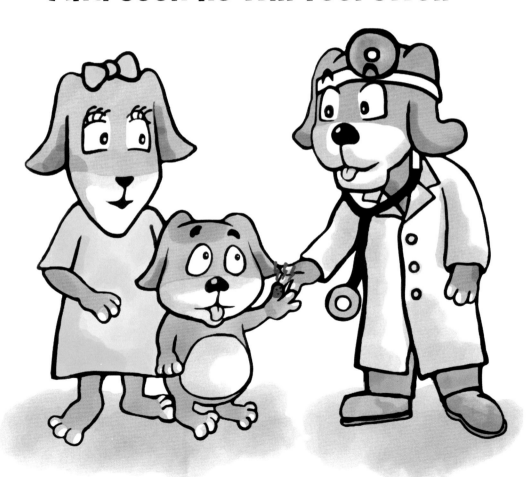

The day before surgery
It's time to eat and drink
Toby finishes his food
His bowl goes in the sink

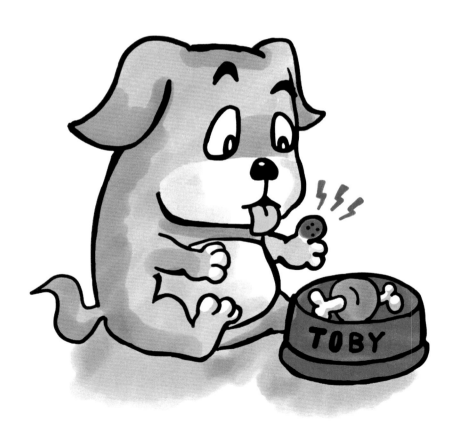

Toby's dad fills the bathtub
He must get squeaky clean
Toby scrubs from head to toe
Soap bubbles fill the scene

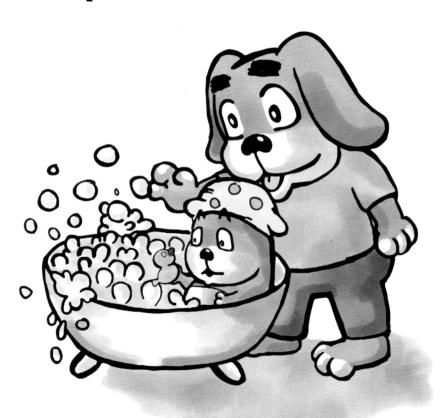

Now it's time to get some rest
Dad says, "Sweet dreams, big guy"
Toby snuggles into bed
And shut his tired eyes

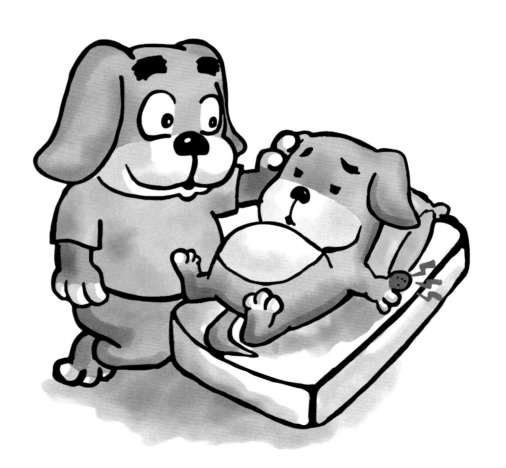

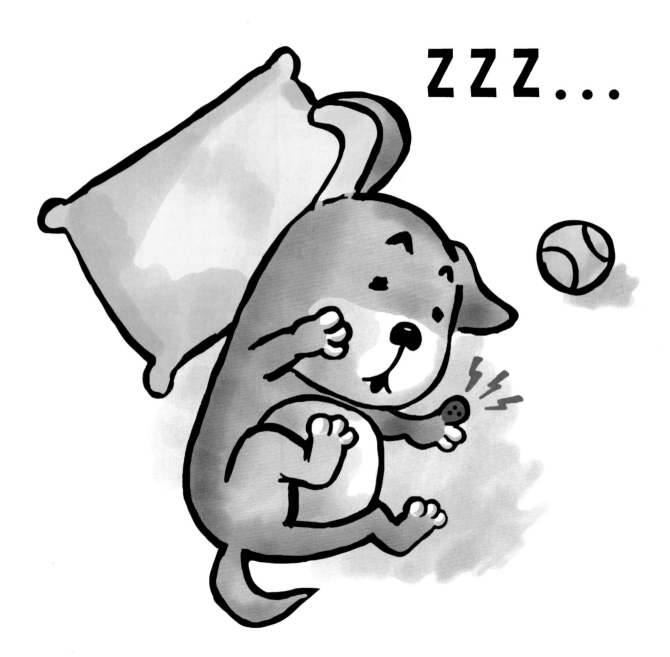

The next day Toby wakes up
And jumps out of his bed
Today is his surgery
He shakes his sleepy head

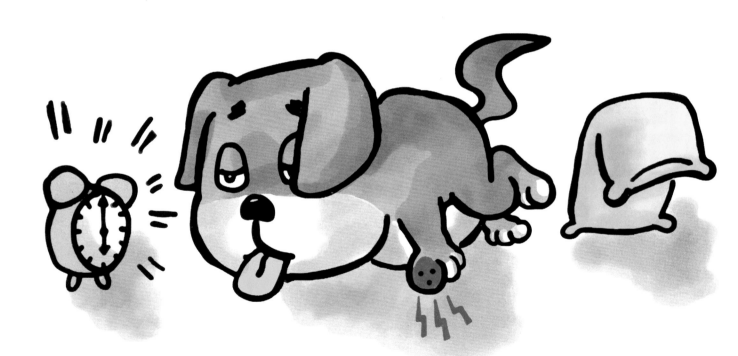

Even though it's breakfast time
He doesn't eat or drink
Toby listens to his Mom
Later he'll have a treat

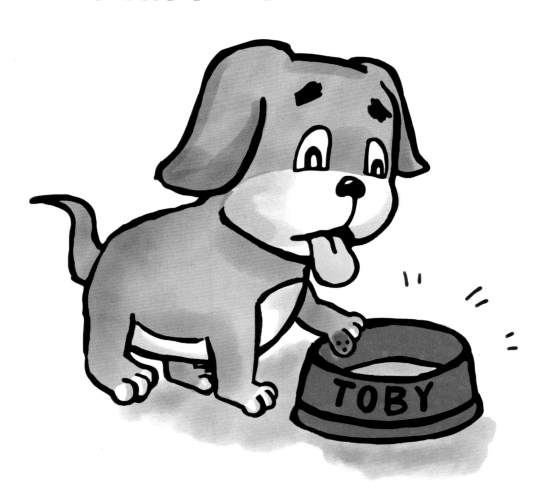

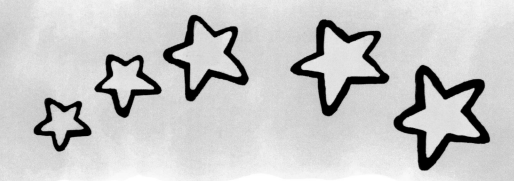

They enter the hospital
Bright pictures fill the walls
Toby looks at all the art
He even spots some balls

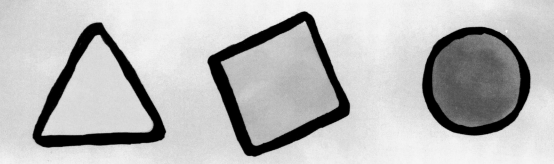

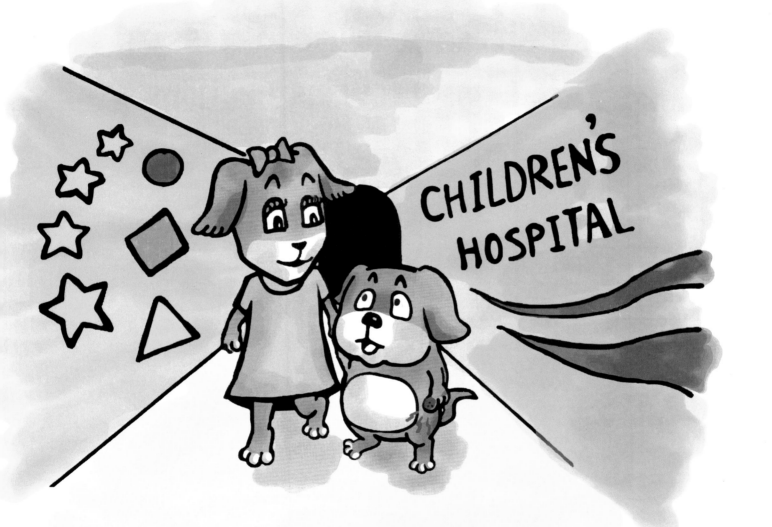

Toby and Mom meet the nurse
She says hello and grins
She has a few instructions
Before they can begin

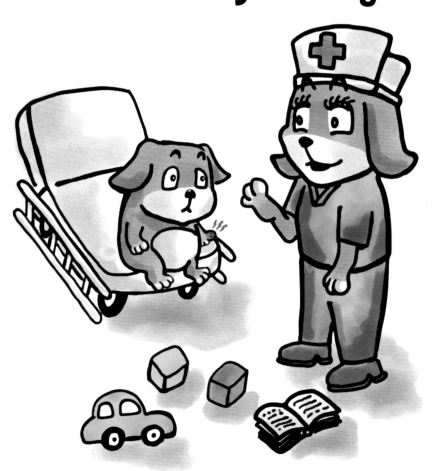

She says it's time for Toby
To change into a gown
It has two strings on the back
Mom helps him tie them down

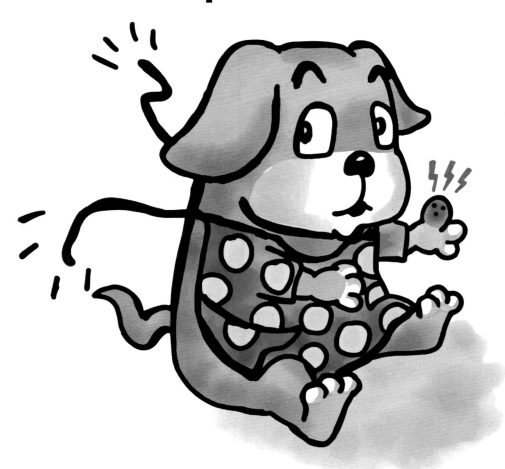

The doctor says good morning
He has a special tool
Toby breathes while he listens
The stethoscope feels cool

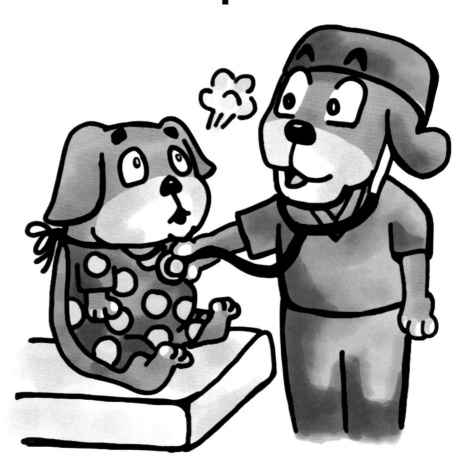

Toby gets a magic mask
Over his mouth and nose
The nurse makes sure it fits
And shows him how it goes

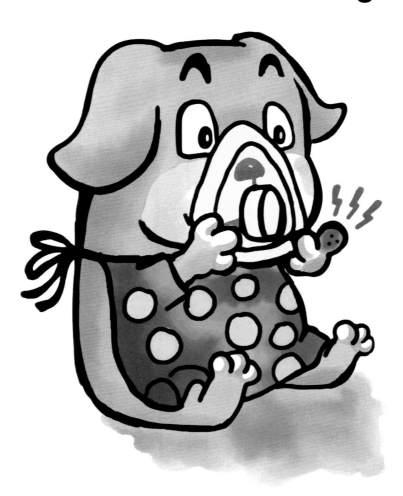

The magic mask smells so good
That Toby wants to share
The doctor says it's special
And just for him to wear

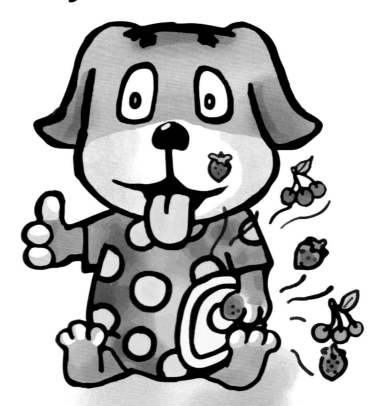

Toby hops on a soft cart
It's time for a short ride
They wheel Toby down the hall
He keeps his paws inside

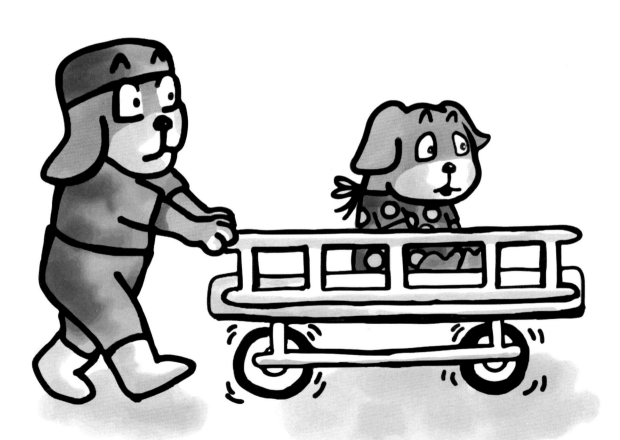

Toby climbs on a new bed
It can move up and down
The doctor smells the mask first
He's silly like a clown

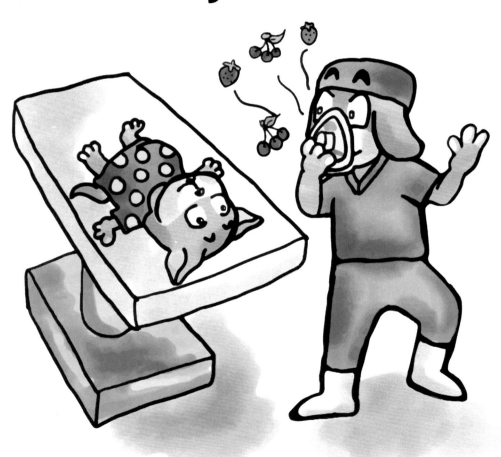

Toby takes a deep breath in
Counting, "One, two and three"
Everyone is smiling now
As Toby goes to sleep

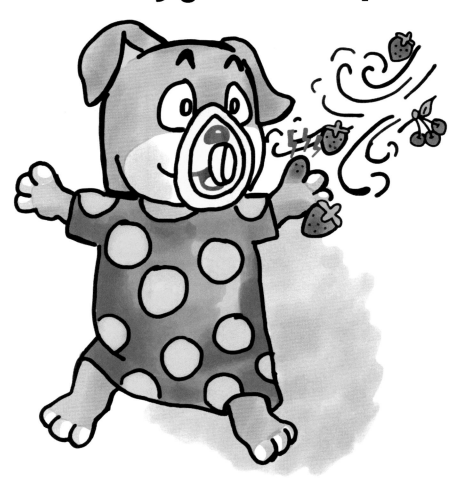

Zzz...

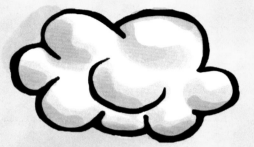

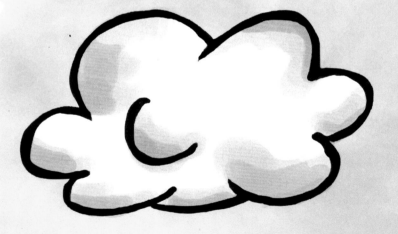

Zzz...

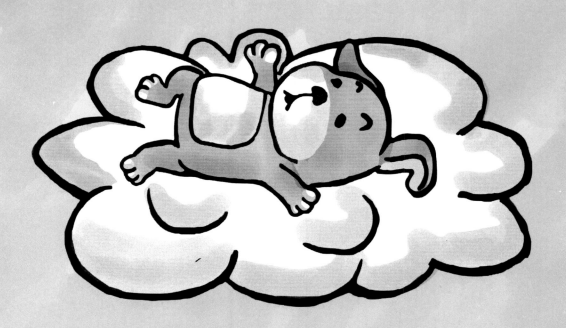

When Toby wakes up later
The surgery's all done
Toby's paw no longer hurts
He's ready for some fun!

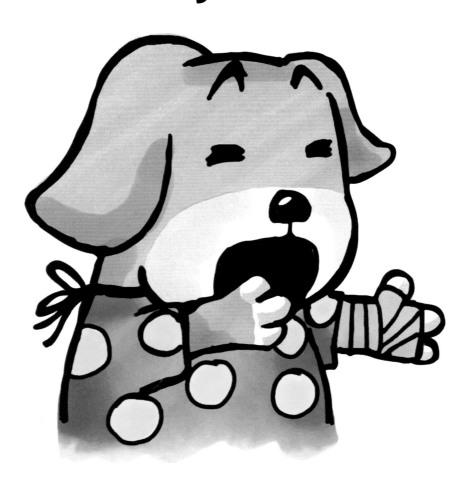

"What happened to my boo boo?"
"Toby, it's gone at last"
He looks down and sees instead
A brightly colored cast

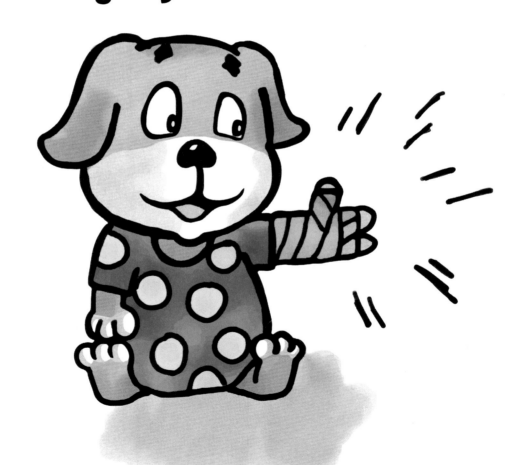

"It's time to go home", Mom says
"We're all so proud of you
You were a very brave boy
And soon you'll feel brand new"

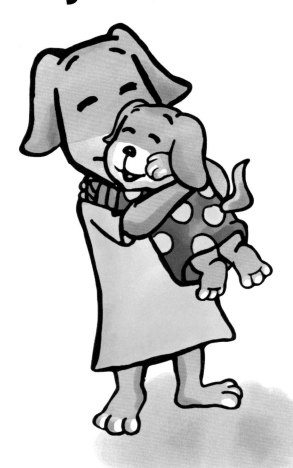

Toby says thank you to all
Who cared for him today
Toby waves goodbye and cheers,
"Now let's go home and play!"

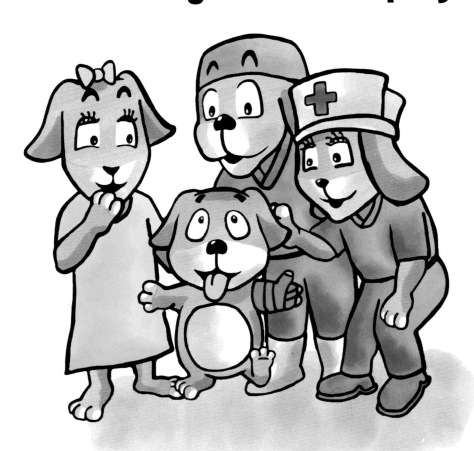

The End

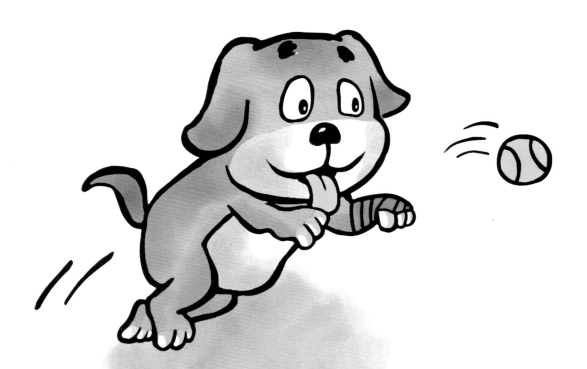

Made in the USA
Middletown, DE
29 March 2019